First Printing: 2019
30 Days of Mindful Health

ISBN: 9781796777482

The Moon Phases Me
Talent, Oregon 97540

@TheMoonPhasesMe on Instagram
MoonPhasesMe@Yahoo.com

Welcome to 30 Days of Mindful Health!

You can use this as a 30 day planner with any program that you are currently on or intend to start. Or you can use this journal as your baby steps to ease into the practice of focusing on your goals and intentions every day.

The top portions are for you to fill in with other goals or daily notes or gratitude. The affirmations are to help you with your new truths. I recommend you rewrite them in your own handwriting every day and repeat them as often as you need to stop and reverse the negative, compulsive thoughts.

If you're taking baby steps, use the next spaces to see what happens if you commit to doing something different with your diet and body for 30 days. The space can also be used to keep your program interesting by changing three things you do each day.

Although it is important not to ignore the negative, for this journal's purpose, the next space is to record all the healthy choices you made without focus on the unhealthy. You don't need to write that you had to use your favorite salad dressing to choke down fresh vegetables unless you're proud of your low fat dressing option. Celebrate eating those veggies regardless!

Write out some things you'd like to try to do different for 30 days:

____________________   ____________________

____________________   ____________________

____________________   ____________________

____________________   ____________________

The law of attraction and other laws of the Universe are true and active whether you are familiar with them or not. I encourage you to look into these laws and how you can make them work for you to reach your goals. This journal is meant to inspire you to talk to yourself differently and to encourage you to ask yourself different questions to help you get started with these laws.

If any of the journal prompts don't resonate with you, feel free to cross out the words and use the space to write other thoughts or track more progress.

There is no magic formula and only you can guarantee the success of the outcome. You probably already know what will happen if you work on some pages for a day or two and then forget about your original intent. Your mind will find ways to distract you and encourage you to procrastinate or go back to old rituals. You might convince yourself that you're bored and feel like you want to just give up and move on to something else. Your mind would much rather stay with the familiar where it thinks life is safe and easier and already knows what will happen; good or bad. *30 Days of Mindful Health* is an opportunity for you to take each day one at a time and find out what happens at the end.

Reasons why I should complete this journal to the end

____

____

____

____

Thoughts, Feelings, Things you want to remember, messages to yourself before you start day 1:

Day 1 ________

Everything I eat nourishes my body.

I love my body.

My health is important to me.

Every move I make burns calories and tones my muscles.

How I plan to eat today:

1.__________________

2.__________________

3.__________________

How I plan to move my body:

1.__________________

2.__________________

3.__________________

Healthy choices I made today:

What will really happen to your mind, body, and soul when you reach the end of your big dream goal?   How will your life be truly different in all these areas?
MIND - How will you think and feel different?

BODY - What are all the ways your body will be different?

SOUL - How will reaching your goal fulfill you?

Other thoughts on how your life will be different at the end of
your goal.

Day 2 _______________

I am beautiful

I have perfect vision.

My hair grows strong and healthy.

I know what I need to do to be healthy.

How I plan to eat today:

1._______________________

2._______________________

3._______________________

How I plan to move my body:

1._______________________

2._______________________

3._______________________

Healthy choices I made today:

If you woke up tomorrow at the end of your goal?   How would
you behave different from morning to night?   Would you eat
different?   Dress different?   Go different places?   Talk to
different people?

What are some of those things that you can begin to do
now?   How can you prepare your life now for the end of your
goal?   What new habits can you begin to create now that
would guarantee your successful outcome?

____
____
____
____
____
____
____
____
____
____
____
____
____
____
____
____
____
____
____
____
____
____
____
____
____
____
____

Day 3 _______

I am strong.

I am full of energy.

My heart is pure.

I am motivated to reach my goals.

How I plan to eat today:

1.______________________

2.______________________

3.______________________

How I plan to move my body:

1.______________________

2.______________________

3.______________________

Healthy choices I made today:

Law of attraction gives us the opportunity to spiral up or spiral down depending on how long we allow ourselves to stay in our low motivation days. On days when you aren't feeling motivated, you don't have to try to get yourself to feel great to gain momentum. You simply need to try to feel better. Use these early, high motivation days to write yourself little notes or make a 'rainy day' playlist. How can you set yourself up for success?

Day 4 _________

I am worthy of a healthy body.

My skin is clear and healthy.

My teeth are strong and white.

I claim good health.

How I plan to eat today:

1.______________________

2.______________________

3.______________________

How I plan to move my body:

1.______________________

2.______________________

3.______________________

Healthy choices I made today:

Who else might be affected by the outcome of your goal?   If you look, feel, and act differently, who might have to adjust?   Are you allowing anyone else to keep you from reaching your goal?

Day 5 _______________

I am loved for who I am.

I love my authentic self.

I value and respect my body.

I know how to take care of my needs.

How I plan to eat today:

1.___________________

2.___________________

3.___________________

How I plan to move my body:

1.___________________

2.___________________

3.___________________

Healthy choices I made today:

What are all the amazing things you love about you right now?

Day 6 ________

I embrace who I am.

I am grateful for the joy of being me.

I direct my own life.

I give myself permission to release extra weight and burdens.

How I plan to eat today:

1.___________________

2.___________________

3.___________________

How I plan to move my body:

1.___________________

2.___________________

3.___________________

Healthy choices I made today:

Do you need to forgive someone for judging you or hurting your feelings?   Are you holding on to a painful memory when your feelings where deeply hurt by someone else that you need to let go?

Do you need to take some time to send some love and forgive yourself for the times when you judged and hurt your own feelings?

Day 7 ________

I embrace change.

I am committed to my health.

I choose the best for me.

I am motivated to continue until I reach my goals.

How I plan to eat today:

1.__________________

2.__________________

3.__________________

How I plan to move my body:

1.__________________

2.__________________

3.__________________

Healthy choices I made today:

How can you change your surroundings to help you align with your goals?   Is it time to put up new pictures around where you work and live?   Do you need to update your closet?   Are you keeping something in your eyeline to remind you of past failures?   What would you be surrounded with if you were already at the end of your goal?

Day 8 _______

I deserve my dream life.

I love myself deeply.

Health is my choice.

I easily accomplish my goals.

<table>
<tr><td>

How I plan to eat today:

1.______________________

2.______________________

3.______________________

</td><td>

How I plan to move my body:

1.______________________

2.______________________

3.______________________

</td></tr>
</table>

Healthy choices I made today:

What activities no longer bring value to your new life? What habits do you need to consider and replace with new, healthier habits?

Day 9 _______________

My wants and needs are important.

I am open to new adventures.

My body is unique and beautiful.

I celebrate my good choices every day.

How I plan to eat today:

1._______________________

2._______________________

3._______________________

How I plan to move my body:

1._______________________

2._______________________

3._______________________

Healthy choices I made today:

What do you wish you knew how to do or want to learn someday?   If time or money were no issue, what would you want to learn more about?

Which of the things that you want to learn will require only a simple internet search?   Which can you order or download a book for?   Are there courses available to you that you can take?   You don't have to do all of them all at once.   Are there any that interest you now to help you reach your goal with new healthy habits?

____
____
____
____
____
____
____
____
____
____
____
____
____
____
____
____
____
____
____
____
____
____
____
____
____
____
____
____
____

Day 10 _______

I trust myself.

I love healthy foods.

I have plenty of energy to exercise.

I honor my life by taking care of my body.

How I plan to eat today:

1.______________________

2.______________________

3.______________________

How I plan to move my body:

1.______________________

2.______________________

3.______________________

Healthy choices I made today:

35 Things you are grateful for right now.

2.____
3.____
4.____
5.____
6.____
7.____
8.____
9.____
10.____
11.____
12.____
13.____
14.____
15.____
16.____
17.____
18.____
19.____
20.____
21.____
22.____
23.____
24.____
25.____
26.____
27.____
28.____
29.____
30.____
31.____
32.____
33.____
34.____
35.____

Day 11 _______

I crave fresh fruits and vegetables.

I have fun with my life.

I am focused.

I have enough energy to do the things I want.

How I plan to eat today:

1.___________________

2.___________________

3.___________________

How I plan to move my body:

1.___________________

2.___________________

3.___________________

Healthy choices I made today:

Has your current condition become a part of your personality that you're afraid to lose? How has your current condition kept you safe? How will people expect you to behave differently after you reach your goal?

Day 12 _______

I am driven.

I believe in myself.

My good health benefits everyone.

Living healthy is easy for me.

How I plan to eat today:

1.______________________

2.______________________

3.______________________

How I plan to move my body:

1.______________________

2.______________________

3.______________________

Healthy choices I made today:

What do you want people to say about you?

Day 13 ________

I am responsible for my own health.

I serve myself well.

I know how to set healthy boundaries.

I know what I need to do to be successful.

How I plan to eat today:

1.________________

2.________________

3.________________

How I plan to move my body:

1.________________

2.________________

3.________________

Healthy choices I made today:

Is there anything you can add to your routine that might give you
a boost toward your goal? What can you do today to get you
closer to your goal?   Write them all out even if you don't intend
to carry them out today. You might find some you'd like to carry
out on another day.

Day 14 ________

When I lose weight I keep it off.

My emotions are well balanced.

I am open to my highest joy.

I have the power to create the body I want.

How I plan to eat today:

1.__________________

2.__________________

3.__________________

How I plan to move my body:

1.__________________

2.__________________

3.__________________

Healthy choices I made today:

Does any part of you fear reaching your goal? Write to any of the parts that tell you that you're goal isn't meant for you or that reaching your goal would make your life more complicated.

Day 15 ________

I am aware of my thoughts and feelings.

I am motivated to take care of myself.

I have unlimited potential.

I am transforming my life for a higher purpose.

How I plan to eat today:

1._______________________

2._______________________

3._______________________

How I plan to move my body:

1._______________________

2._______________________

3._______________________

Healthy choices I made today:

Write affirmations how you want to live in your body from head to toe. ("My hair grows long and healthy"; "My teeth are strong and white.";   "My vision is perfect") Incorporate these in your daily self talk. Find your favorites and use them as Mantras to redirect any negative thoughts that creep in.

Day 16 ________

I am overflowing with joy.

My life is in my control.

I am worthy of respect.

I welcome miracles into my life.

How I plan to eat today:

1.____________________

2.____________________

3.____________________

How I plan to move my body:

1.____________________

2.____________________

3.____________________

Healthy choices I made today:

What habits are you still holding onto that keep you stuck? How are these habits still serving you? What will it feel like to release these habits after you feel through the initial discomfort?

Day 17 _______

I celebrate every day.

I have the courage to live my dreams.

I am responsible.

My strengths are greater than my struggles.

How I plan to eat today:

1. _______________

2. _______________

3. _______________

How I plan to move my body:

1. _______________

2. _______________

3. _______________

Healthy choices I made today:

How do you feel about the progress you've made so far? Have you amended your original goals to allow success or to accept failure? Is now a time that you need to catch up or can you relax and enjoy your progress?

Day 18 _________

I am living my best life now.

My heart is filled with gratitude.

I am blessed.

I am devoted to my dream life.

How I plan to eat today:

1.___________________

2.___________________

3.___________________

How I plan to move my body:

1.___________________

2.___________________

3.___________________

Healthy choices I made today:

Are you waiting for someone to rescue you? Does any part of your goal rely on someone else? What can you do or learn how to do that you have been relying on from someone else?

Day 19 ________

I feel strong.

I feel connected.

I know the best path for my life.

I appreciate my good health.

How I plan to eat today:

1.____________________

2.____________________

3.____________________

How I plan to move my body:

1.____________________

2.____________________

3.____________________

Healthy choices I made today:

How have you changed in the past couple of weeks?   What have you learned about yourself?

Day 20 _________

I always attract fun into my life.

I deserve to be in the best health.

I have amazing luck.

My health is important to me.

How I plan to eat today:

1.___________________

2.___________________

3.___________________

How I plan to move my body:

1.___________________

2.___________________

3.___________________

Healthy choices I made today:

If you had all the time you needed to do anything you wanted,
what would you do? Where would you go?   Who would you
contact or spend time with?   What would you finish?

How can you find the time to start creating new habits by replacing old habits? Can you turn the TV off earlier in the evening and wake up earlier to get more done? Can you make coffee at home instead of getting one at a shop on the way to work so that you have ten minutes to meditate?

Day 21 _______

I have unlimited potential.

My self worth is constantly growing.

I am excited about my life.

Success follows me everywhere.

How I plan to eat today:

1.______________________

2.______________________

3.______________________

How I plan to move my body:

1.______________________

2.______________________

3.______________________

Healthy choices I made today:

Do you believe that you deserve to be in the perfect health at
the perfect weight?

____

____

____

____

____

____

____

____

____

____

____

____

____

____

____

____

____

____

____

____

____

____

Do you believe that you deserve to be in the perfect health at
the perfect weight?

____

____

____

____

Day 22 _______

I am an unstoppable force.

I recognize my own beauty.

My positive thoughts lead to success.

I achieve whatever I desire.

How I plan to eat today:

1. _______________

2. _______________

3. _______________

How I plan to move my body:

1. _______________

2. _______________

3. _______________

Healthy choices I made today:

What are ways you are still resisting the outcome of your goals?
Are you sabotaging your progress in any way?

Day 23 _______

I was born for greatness.

I radiate love and happiness.

I speak kindly of others.

I make great decisions.

How I plan to eat today:

1._______________________

2._______________________

3._______________________

How I plan to move my body:

1._______________________

2._______________________

3._______________________

Healthy choices I made today:

If you chose to start over at day one today, what would you do differently?

Day 24 _______

I am surrounded with love.

I have faith in myself.

I am proud of who I am.

All is well.

How I plan to eat today:

1.______________________

2.______________________

3.______________________

How I plan to move my body:

1.______________________

2.______________________

3.______________________

Healthy choices I made today:

Is fear of not reaching your goals keeping you from being more effecting at reaching for them?

Day 25 __________

I trust myself.

I have the drive to reach my goals.

I know what I want.

I take inspired action.

How I plan to eat today:

1._______________________

2._______________________

3._______________________

How I plan to move my body:

1._______________________

2._______________________

3._______________________

Healthy choices I made today:

How has focusing on your goals every day gotten you closer to where you want to be?

Day 26 ________

I love my healthy lifestyle.

I believe in myself.

Living healthy is easy for me.

I serve myself well.

How I plan to eat today:

1._______________

2._______________

3._______________

How I plan to move my body:

1._______________

2._______________

3._______________

Healthy choices I made today:

Which goals do you need to carry through to the next phase?
What goals are still important to you?

____
____

____
____

____
____

____
____

____
____

____
____

____
____

____
____

____
____

____
____

Day 27 ________

Life is good.

I follow my true bliss.

My dream life is my priority.

I focus on what is important to me.

How I plan to eat today:

1.___________________

2.___________________

3.___________________

How I plan to move my body:

1.___________________

2.___________________

3.___________________

Healthy choices I made today:

What fun goals can you set for yourself in all other areas of
your life?   When you think of big dreams that might take a year
or more, break them down into what you can accomplish in 30
days.   Write as many as you can think of and choose a few at
a time to work on.

Day 28 _______

I deserve the best.

I am strong.

I let go of past hurts.

I always sleep restfully.

How I plan to eat today:

1.______________________

2.______________________

3.______________________

How I plan to move my body:

1.______________________

2.______________________

3.______________________

Healthy choices I made today:

Write a list of things that you'd like to try to do every day for 30 days just to see what would happen.

Day 29 _______

I choose to be healthy.

My life is beautiful.

My body is strong.

I love who I am becoming.

How I plan to eat today:

1.______________________

2.______________________

3.______________________

How I plan to move my body:

1.______________________

2.______________________

3.______________________

Healthy choices I made today:

Write out everything that you've accomplished, learned, manifested and can be proud of from the last 29 days.

Day 30 _______

I am filled with positive energy.

I am healthier than ever.

I am full of confidence.

I wake up with a peaceful mind.

How I plan to eat today:

1.____________________

2.____________________

3.____________________

How I plan to move my body:

1.____________________

2.____________________

3.____________________

Healthy choices I made today:

Write out how you'd like for the next 30 days to go.

Write out how you'd like for the next 30 days to go.

9 781796 777482